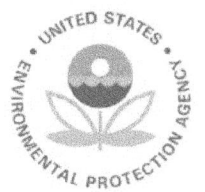 U.S. ENVIRONMENTAL PROTECTION AGENCY
OFFICE OF INSPECTOR GENERAL

Catalyst for Improving the Environment

Hotline Report

Revisions Needed to National Contingency Plan Based on Deepwater Horizon Oil Spill

Report No. 11-P-0534

August 25, 2011

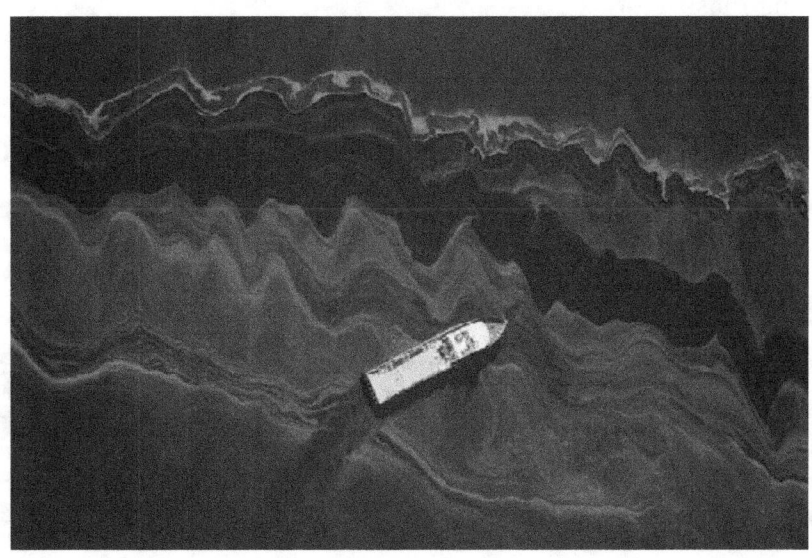

Report Contributors:

Patrick Gilbride
Erin Barnes-Weaver
Todd Goldman
Mary Anne Strasser
Stephanie Wake
Susan Charen

Abbreviations

BFT	Baffled Flask Test
CWA	Clean Water Act
EPA	U.S. Environmental Protection Agency
FOSC	Federal On-Scene Coordinator
NCP	National Oil and Hazardous Substances Pollution Contingency Plan, also known as the National Contingency Plan
NRT	National Response Team
OEM	Office of Emergency Management
OIG	Office of Inspector General
OPA	Oil Pollution Act
ORD	Office of Research and Development
OSC	On-Scene Coordinator
OSWER	Office of Solid Waste and Emergency Response
RRT	Regional Response Team
SFT	Swirling Flask Test
USCG	U.S. Coast Guard

Cover photo: An overhead view of the Deepwater Horizon oil spill. (U.S. Coast Guard photo)

At a Glance

Catalyst for Improving the Environment

Why We Did This Review

The U.S. Environmental Protection Agency (EPA), Office of Inspector General (OIG), received two Hotline complaints on the use of dispersants in response to the Deepwater Horizon oil spill in the Gulf of Mexico. We reviewed the steps EPA took to analyze the dispersant Corexit for inclusion on the National Contingency Plan (NCP) Product Schedule. We also determined EPA's role in the decision to use Corexit in the response. The OIG Office of Counsel addressed a perjury allegation in one complaint.

Background

The NCP establishes national response capability and coordination for oil spills. The NCP Product Schedule lists spill-mitigating chemicals that responders can use in carrying out the NCP, including dispersants that emulsify, disperse, or solubilize oil into the water column.

For further information, contact our Office of Congressional, Public Affairs, and Management at (202) 566-2391.

The full report is at:
www.epa.gov/oig/reports/2011/
20110825-11-P-0534.pdf

Revisions Needed to National Contingency Plan Based on Deepwater Horizon Oil Spill

What We Found

EPA and the manufacturer of Corexit completed required steps to include Corexit products on the NCP Product Schedule. However, EPA has not updated the NCP since 1994 to include the most appropriate efficacy testing protocol. Subpart J of the NCP identifies requirements a manufacturer must meet to include a product on the Product Schedule, including efficacy results using the Swirling Flask Test. EPA has considered revising Subpart J to change efficacy testing procedures to the more reproducible Baffled Flask Test. However, EPA had not finalized the rulemaking before the Deepwater Horizon oil spill occurred because of competing priorities and changes in management. If EPA had updated Subpart J, more reliable efficacy data may have been available during the oil spill.

Responders to the Deepwater Horizon oil spill could have used other dispersants, but not within the applicable window of time designated by Addendum 2 to a directive issued by EPA and the Coast Guard. EPA's involvement in the response included issuing Joint Directives to BP, making operational decisions, and conducting additional dispersant testing. EPA involved senior officials in the response because (a) the Agency was not prepared for the unprecedented volume and duration of dispersant use and subsea application, and (b) additional clarity was needed on roles and responsibilities in responding to a Spill of National Significance. The involvement of senior EPA officials created confusion as to who at EPA led response efforts for dispersant use.

The OIG Office of Counsel did not find evidence supporting the perjury allegation.

We noted that EPA took proactive actions to make health and environmental data available on the Agency's website throughout the spill response. Also, EPA demonstrated proactive efforts to improve emergency response plans.

What We Recommend

We recommend that the Office of Solid Waste and Emergency Response establish policies to review and update contingency plans incorporating lessons learned during the Deepwater Horizon oil spill, and clarify roles and responsibilities for Spills of National Significance. We also recommend that the office take steps to revise Subpart J to incorporate the most appropriate efficacy testing protocol and capture dispersant information. We recommend that the Office of Research and Development develop a research plan on long-term health and environmental effects of dispersants. The Agency generally agreed with our recommendations.

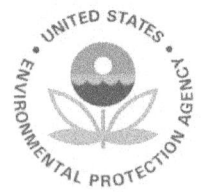

UNITED STATES ENVIRONMENTAL PROTECTION AGENCY
WASHINGTON, D.C. 20460

August 25, 2011

MEMORANDUM

SUBJECT: Revisions Needed to National Contingency Plan Based on
Deepwater Horizon Oil Spill
Report No. 11-P-0534

FROM: Arthur A. Elkins, Jr.
Inspector General

TO: Mathy Stanislaus
Assistant Administrator for Solid Waste and Emergency Response

Paul Anastas
Assistant Administrator for Research and Development

This is our report on the subject audit conducted by the Office of Inspector General (OIG) of the U.S. Environmental Protection Agency (EPA). This report contains findings that describe problems we identified and corrective actions we recommend. This report represents the opinion of the OIG and does not necessarily represent the final EPA position. EPA managers will make final determinations on matters in this report in accordance with established audit resolution procedures.

The estimated direct labor and travel costs for this report are $277,478.

Action Required

In accordance with EPA Manual 2750, you are required to provide a written response to this report within 90 calendar days. You should include a corrective actions plan for agreed-upon actions, including milestone dates. We will post your response on the OIG's public website, along with our memorandum commenting on your response. Please provide your response as an Adobe PDF file that complies with the accessibility requirements of Section 508 of the Rehabilitation Act of 1973, as amended. The final response should not contain data that you do not want released to the public; if your response contains such data, you should identify the data for redaction or removal. We have no objections to the further release of this report to the public. We will post this report to our website at http://www.epa.gov/oig.

If you or your staff have any questions regarding this report, please contact Melissa Heist, Assistant Inspector General for Audit, at (202) 566-0899 or Heist.Melissa@epa.gov; or Patrick Gilbride, Director, at (303) 312-6969 or Gilbride.Patrick@epa.gov.

Table of Contents

Chapters

Appendices

Chapter 1
Introduction

Purpose

The U.S. Environmental Protection Agency (EPA), Office of Inspector General (OIG), received two separate Hotline complaints regarding the use of dispersants in response to the Deepwater Horizon oil spill in the Gulf of Mexico. The first, received on May 16, 2010, alleged that EPA "approved" the use of Corexit although there were other less harmful substances available. We used the following objectives to address the first Hotline complaint:

- Determine what steps EPA took to analyze Corexit to include it on the National Contingency Plan Product Schedule.

- Determine EPA's role in the decision to use Corexit over other dispersants in the Deepwater Horizon oil spill.

The second Hotline complaint, received July 25, 2010, alleged that EPA was covering up the effects of the dispersant being used and alluded to EPA staff lying and committing perjury. The OIG Office of Counsel reviewed the perjury allegation.

Background

EPA's Oil Response Authorities and Organization

EPA's Office of Solid Waste and Emergency Response (OSWER) provides policy, guidance, and direction for the Agency's emergency response and waste programs. Within OSWER, the Office of Emergency Management (OEM) works with other federal partners to prevent accidents as well as to maintain superior response capabilities. While several laws address EPA's emergency management program, two laws set forth EPA's responsibilities for responses to oil spills:

- Federal Water Pollution Control Act, as amended (Clean Water Act, or CWA)
- Oil Pollution Act (OPA) of 1990

The CWA is the principal federal statute protecting navigable waters and adjoining shorelines from pollution. Section 311 of the CWA addresses pollution from oil and hazardous substance releases, providing EPA and the U.S. Coast Guard (USCG) the authority to establish a program for preventing, preparing for, and responding to oil spills. EPA implements CWA provisions through a variety of regulations, including the National Oil and Hazardous Substances Pollution Contingency Plan (National Contingency Plan, or NCP).

OPA, which expanded the federal government's ability to respond to oil spills, became federal law following the Exxon Valdez oil spill. OPA provided new requirements for contingency planning by both government and industry. OPA also established a 13-member Interagency Coordinating Committee on Oil Pollution Research, currently chaired by the USCG. Executive Order 12777, signed in 1991, implemented OPA and delegated responsibilities under Section 311 of CWA to EPA, the U.S. Department of the Interior, and the U.S. Department of Transportation.

National Contingency Plan

The NCP serves as the federal government's blueprint for responding to oil spills and hazardous substance releases. The NCP established national response capability and overall coordination among the hierarchy of responders and contingency plans for oil spills and hazardous substance releases, including a Spill of National Significance. For discharges occurring in the coastal zone, the USCG Commandant can designate a spill as a Spill of National Significance due to its severity, size, location, actual or potential impact on the public health and welfare or the environment, or the complexity of the necessary response effort. The federal government performs three fundamental activities pursuant to the NCP:

- Preparedness planning and coordination for response to a discharge of oil or release of a hazardous substance, pollutant, or contaminant
- Notification and communications
- Response operations at the scene of a discharge or release

The NCP is a key component of the National Response System, a multilayered response network of individuals and teams from federal, state, local, and tribal agencies, and industry. The system includes: the National Response Center, On-Scene Coordinators (OSCs), the National Response Team (NRT), and the Regional Response Teams (RRTs). The NCP designates EPA and USCG roles and responsibilities for the NRT, RRTs, and OSCs. The NRT is responsible for national response and preparedness planning, coordinating regional planning, and providing policy guidance and support to RRTs. The Director for OEM serves as EPA's representative/chair to the NRT; the USCG serves as vice-chair. RRTs are responsible for regional planning and preparedness activities, and providing advice and support to the OSC when activated during a response. The RRTs are co-chaired by EPA and the USCG.

The NCP designates the USCG as the lead response agency and appoints the OSC for spills within or threatening coastal zones, whereas EPA leads and appoints the OSC for response to spills that occur in inland zones. For a Spill of National Significance in the coastal zone, the NCP states that the USCG may name a National Incident Commander to assume the role of OSC in communicating with affected parties and the public, and coordinating federal, state, local, and international resources at the national level. For a Spill of National Significance in the inland zone, the EPA Administrator may name a senior Agency official to assist the OSC. The NCP says coordination will involve, as appropriate, the NRT, RRTs, governors of affected states, and mayors or other chief executives of local governments.

The NCP outlines requirements for contingency planning under OPA and requires the development of Regional and Area Contingency Plans to prepare for the possibility of an oil spill or hazardous substance release. Area Contingency Plans, when implemented in conjunction with other provisions of the NCP, must be adequate to remove a worst-case discharge and to mitigate or prevent a substantial threat of such a discharge.

NCP Product Schedule

Executive Order 12777 delegated to EPA's Administrator the functions in CWA Section 311 on schedules of dispersants. Subpart J of the NCP requires EPA to prepare and maintain the Product Schedule, which OEM maintains. The schedule is a list of dispersants and other spill-mitigating devices that may be used in carrying out the NCP. Dispersants are chemicals that accelerate the natural dispersion process created by energy, allowing oil to mix with water. Dispersants include surfactants that break down oil into smaller droplets that are more likely to dissolve into the water column. The decision to use dispersants involves trade-offs between decreasing risks to water surface and shoreline habitats, and increasing potential risks to organisms in the water column and on the sea floor.

Subpart J lists 12 data requirements that manufacturers must submit to have EPA consider including their dispersant products on the schedule. These requirements include dispersant application and storage methods, and efficacy and toxicity testing information. The requirements limit toxicity testing to acute (short-term) studies on one fish species and one shrimp species. Dispersants must demonstrate at least a 50 percent plus or minus 5 percent effectiveness on the average of two crude oils using a Swirling Flask Test (meaning the product must disperse at least 45 percent of oil in testing). Subpart J requires that laboratories conduct efficacy and toxicity testing and manufacturers submit test results from these laboratories with their product information. There are two levels of review for what manufacturers submit: one performed by an EPA contractor, and one performed by an OEM Product Schedule Manager who reviews materials and data for completeness before listing products on the schedule. EPA does not perform product testing to independently confirm test results submitted by manufacturers.

Inclusion on the Product Schedule does not mean that EPA approved the product for use. Instead, it means the product may be authorized for use during a spill response by the designated federal OSC.

Deepwater Horizon Oil Spill

The Deepwater Horizon mobile offshore drilling unit, owned and managed by Transocean and contracted by BP p.l.c., began drilling operations in January 2010. On April 20, 2010, the Deepwater Horizon unit exploded and caught fire, and on April 22 it sank. The spill lasted 87 days and spilled an estimated 4.9 million barrels of oil,[1] making it the largest marine oil spill in U.S. history. The USCG, as designated federal OSC (FOSC) for spills occurring in the coastal zone, led the federal response to the spill. On April 29, 2010, the Secretary of the Department of Homeland Security designated the spill as a Spill of National Significance and on May 1, 2010, named a USCG Admiral (then Commandant) as National Incident Commander.

Responders first used dispersants on April 22. Responders used Corexit EC9527A and Corexit EC9500A during the response. The standing inventory of EC9527A was depleted, and EC9500A became the primary dispersant used during the response. On April 30, BP suggested using dispersants subsurface at the source of the spill, a novel approach to oil spill mitigation. Responders hoped that, in addition to reducing shoreline impacts, subsurface application would result in less dispersants used overall. BP conducted three rounds of testing between April 30 and May 10 on subsurface application, and a mix of federal scientists (including but not limited to EPA, the USCG, and the National Oceanic and Atmospheric Administration) worked to create a monitoring protocol for subsurface dispersant use. Table 1 lists major response events, including joint actions of EPA and the USCG on dispersant applications (denoted in red).

---

[1] In its response to our draft report, OSWER indicated that there is an ongoing investigation into the number of barrels spilled.

Table 1: Major events in the Deepwater Horizon oil spill response

Date	Event
04/20/10	Deepwater Horizon oil drilling rig exploded.
04/29/10	Homeland Security Secretary designated the spill as a Spill of National Significance and the USCG appointed a National Incident Commander (on 05/01/10).
05/10/10	EPA and the USCG issued a Joint Directive to BP requiring them to implement a monitoring and assessment plan for subsurface dispersant applications.
05/14/10	EPA and the USCG issue Addendum 1 to the Directive on specific details of the monitoring plan and requiring BP to include a more thorough oil analysis that will allow EPA to determine whether the plume is toxic to aquatic life.
05/20/10	EPA and the USCG issued Addendum 2 to the Directive requiring BP to identify and use a less toxic and as effective dispersant. BP responded to Addendum 2, saying Corexit was the only dispersant available in sufficiently large quantities to be useful at the time of the spill.
05/26/10	EPA and the USCG issued Addendum 3 to the Directive telling BP to establish a goal to reduce dispersant application by 75 percent. The Addendum limited subsurface dispersant application to 15,000 gallons per day, and eliminated surface application altogether except for when an exemption is approved.
06/09/10	EPA Administrator approved a process for daily approval of surface dispersant applications.
06/30/10	EPA issued toxicity results on testing on eight dispersants listed on the NCP Product Schedule. EPA concluded that Corexit EC9500A was not significantly more toxic than other dispersants tested.
07/15/10	The well was capped and oil flow halted.
08/02/10	EPA issued toxicity results on the second round of testing. Results confirmed that the dispersant used in response, Corexit EC9500A, is generally no more or less toxic than other available alternatives.

Source: Information collected by OIG research based on a variety of sources.

Numerous questions have been raised on the effectiveness of dispersants, their inherent toxicity, and the toxicity of dispersed oil. EPA maintains a modest oil spill research and development program with one staff member and limited contract staff support, and a budget between $500,000 and $700,000 annually over the last 10 years.

Noteworthy Achievements

To increase transparency, EPA made health and environmental data available on the Agency's website throughout the spill response and recovery operation. EPA monitored air, water, sediment, and waste generated by the cleanup operations. EPA posted environmental data, including air quality and water samples, on the Agency's website as collected, and updated postings as needed. EPA's monitoring and sampling activities provided the USCG and state and local governments with information on potential impacts of the oil to the human health of residents and aquatic life along the shoreline. EPA's activities included:

- Collecting samples along the shoreline and monitoring for chemicals related to oil and dispersants in the air, water, and sediment
- Supporting and advising USCG efforts to clean the reclaimed oil and waste from the shoreline

- Being actively involved with new monitoring procedures for observing effects of dispersants in the subsurface environment

OSWER demonstrated proactive efforts to improve emergency response plans. In a November 2, 2010, memorandum, the OSWER Assistant Administrator listed interim actions that RRTs should take in order to benefit from the experiences and knowledge gained during the Deepwater Horizon oil spill. The memorandum directed Regional Administrators to engage federal partners through the NRT to reassess dispersant use guidelines under the NCP for future oil spills. The memorandum tasked RRT representatives to work with their partners to revise Area and Regional Contingency Plans with respect to dispersant use. For example, the memorandum said plans should develop or address:

- A hierarchy of preferred oil spill response measures, including mechanical recovery (such as skimming/booming and controlled burning), followed by dispersant use
- Site-specific and oil-specific rationale for environmental trade-offs and favorable dispersant use conditions, such as mixing energy, water depth, wind speed, and distance from shorelines
- Steps to include the public and keep them informed
- A process for longer-term responses and the need for monitoring information to reassess dispersant and chemical use

Since the Deepwater Horizon oil spill, EPA formed a workgroup, which includes OEM, to address necessary revisions to the NCP, and undertook efforts to gather and apply lessons learned from the spill.

Scope and Methodology

We conducted our work from August 2010 to May 2011 in accordance with generally accepted government auditing standards. Those standards require that we plan and perform our review to obtain sufficient, appropriate evidence to provide a reasonable basis for our findings and conclusions based on our objectives. We believe that the evidence obtained provides a reasonable basis for our findings and conclusions based on our objectives.

To address our first objective, we analyzed the NCP Product Schedule and other relevant laws and regulations to determine the steps EPA takes to include a dispersant on the schedule. We reviewed information submitted by the manufacturer of Corexit EC9527A and EC9500A to get those dispersants listed on the schedule.

To address our second objective, we reviewed relevant laws and regulations that authorize the federal government's response to oil spills. We reviewed federal guidance and documents to understand established policies and procedures used throughout the response. We conducted research on dispersants, including dispersant testing protocols and stockpiles. We gathered and analyzed information and conducted interviews with OSWER, OEM, Region 6,[2] the EPA Office of Research and Development (ORD), and the USCG to understand EPA's role in decisionmaking on the use of dispersants. Appendix A provides additional information on our scope and methodology.

The OIG Office of Counsel addressed components of one Hotline complaint pertaining to perjury allegations. Office of Counsel reviewed testimony by EPA senior officials to determine whether evidence demonstrated that perjury existed. Appendix B summarizes Office of Counsel's perjury review results.

---

[2] Responders activated the Region 6 RRT because the Deepwater Horizon oil spill occurred in Region 6 waters.

Chapter 2
EPA Needs to Revise Subpart J of the NCP to Include a More Appropriate Testing Procedure

EPA and the manufacturer of Corexit completed required steps to include both Corexit EC9527A and EC9500A on the NCP Product Schedule. However, EPA has not updated the NCP since 1994 to include the most appropriate efficacy testing protocol. Subpart J of the NCP identifies the requirements a manufacturer must meet for a product's inclusion on the Product Schedule. One of the 12 data requirements is efficacy results using the Swirling Flask Test (SFT). EPA's OEM considered revising Subpart J to include changing the efficacy testing procedure to the Baffled Flask Test (BFT)—a more reproducible testing procedure identified in an EPA study a decade ago. OEM staff worked on revising the rule for a few years, but had not finalized the rulemaking before the Deepwater Horizon spill occurred because of competing priorities and changes in management. Decisionmakers at the time of the spill relied on efficacy results from the SFT, which was found to be susceptible to human error. The BFT has proved more reproducible, and if EPA had updated Subpart J to include it as the standard testing protocol, more reliable efficacy data may have been available at the time of the Deepwater Horizon oil spill.

EPA Could Have Used a Better Testing Procedure

Section 311 of the CWA states that the NCP shall include a schedule identifying dispersants that may be used in carrying out the NCP and the quantities of and waters in which such dispersants may be used safely. NCP Subpart J delegates EPA the responsibility to "prepare a schedule of dispersants, other chemicals, and other spill mitigating devices and substances, if any, that may be used in carrying out the NCP." To include a product on the schedule, a manufacturer must submit 12 data requirements, including efficacy and toxicity testing results obtained from an independent laboratory. At the time of the Deepwater Horizon oil spill, Subpart J included the SFT as the required efficacy testing procedure.

EPA's NCP Product Schedule includes as dispersants Corexit EC9527A and EC9500A, both of which were used in the Deepwater Horizon oil spill response. EPA first listed Corexit EC9527A on March 10, 1978, and Corexit EC9500A on April 13, 1994. The Corexit manufacturer submitted all required data, including SFT results with effectiveness values demonstrating at least 50 percent, plus or minus 5 percent, on the average of two crude oils. (Corexit EC9527A efficacy results equaled 50.4 percent and Corexit EC9500A results equaled 50 percent.) There are two levels of review when manufacturers submit product information for inclusion: one performed by an EPA contractor, and the other performed by EPA's Product Schedule Manager who reviews materials and data for completeness before listing products on the schedule. EPA is not required to perform product testing to confirm test results submitted by manufacturers.

The NCP was revised in 1994 to adopt the SFT as the official efficacy laboratory testing procedure to list a dispersant on the schedule. Multiple EPA and outside experts have expressed concerns with the SFT. In a 2001 report, ORD described how it discovered—soon after the 1994 revision and after the SFT's first year of use—"unexpected large discrepancies" between the data submitted by dispersant manufacturers and those generated by EPA contract laboratories.[3] An ORD scientist and EPA's lead oil spill researcher said SFT procedures are not reproducible and are susceptible to human error. Thus, EPA initiated research in 1999 to determine and correct the cause of the SFT's poor reproducibility.

In November 2001, a group of scientists published an EPA-funded research study introducing a new testing procedure—the BFT—that was found to be more reproducible than the SFT. An ORD scientist explained that a major source of reproducibility problems with the SFT pertained to the flask design, which the new BFT design addressed. Figure 1 shows both designs. In addition, a 2005 National Academy of Sciences report suggested the BFT as a better indicator of efficacy than the SFT. The 2008–2009 biennial report for the Interagency Coordinating Committee on Oil Pollution Research noted that EPA intended for the BFT to be the new standard. A BP representative said that he does not find the SFT relevant in the field.

Figure 1: SFT and BFT designs

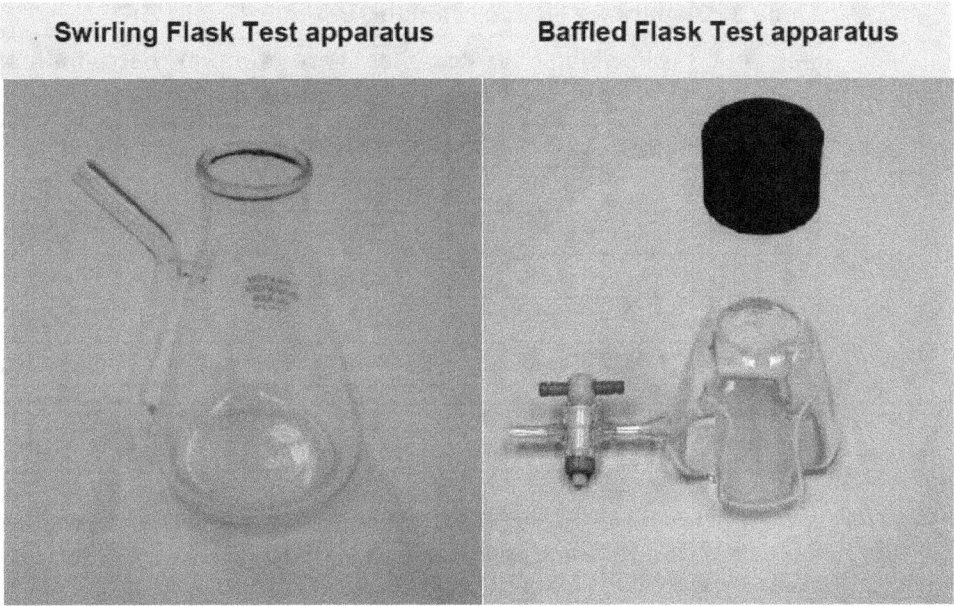

Source: ORD.

---

[3] EPA's lead oil spill researcher, Albert D. Venosa, described this history and early concerns with the SFT in a 2010 report, *Use of the Baffled Flask Test to Determine the Dispersibility of S. Louisiana Crude Oil by Eight Oil Dispersant Products Listed on the NCP Product Schedule.*

Concerns with the SFT were one issue that prompted EPA to consider revising Subpart J when staff first identified issues a decade ago. EPA's OEM informed us it had worked on revising the rule for a few years and "prepared a proposed rule to modify the efficacy test and several other test and data requirements planned for promulgation in late spring 2010. However, publication of the proposed rule was set aside. . . ." Former Agency managers said EPA did not finalize revisions due to changes in management and competing priorities for program resources. EPA promulgated revisions to the Spill Prevention, Control, and Countermeasure rule in 2002 and implementation of the rule became an Agency focus demanding staff and resources. As a result, the NCP has not been updated since 1994.

Since the spill, the EPA Administrator testified that changes are needed to the NCP's Subpart J, including dispersant registration and a more complete range of tests to address human and environmental health. EPA informed us, "the available record does not suggest the dispersant used was ineffective, or that it would not have also passed the BFT." In fact, Corexit EC9500A,[4] whose SFT results rank as the least effective dispersant, is the second most effective dispersant using BFT results. Table 2 lists dispersant efficacy rankings using SFT information from EPA's NCP Product Schedule Technical Notebook and BFT results from ORD's 2010 study. This recent study intended to determine how effective the eight dispersants currently available on the schedule performed on south Louisiana crude oil at the two temperatures in the Gulf of Mexico (5°C represents temperature conditions for the deep sea dispersant injection, and 25°C represents temperature conditions for surface application).

Table 2: Dispersant efficacy ranking using SFT and BFT

	Ranking of efficacy test results (most to least effective)		
	SFT	BFT (5°)	BFT (25°)
1	DISPERSIT SPC 1000	DISPERSIT SPC 1000	DISPERSIT SPC 1000
2	ZI-400	COREXIT EC9500A	COREXIT EC9500A
3	SAF-RON GOLD	JD-2000	JD-2000
4	JD-2000	NOKOMIS 3-F4	ZI-400
5	NOKOMIS 3-AA	NOKOMIS 3-AA	NOKOMIS 3-AA
6	NOKOMIS 3-F4	SAF-RON GOLD	SEA BRAT #4
7	SEA BRAT #4	ZI-400	NOKOMIS 3-F4
8	COREXIT EC9500A	SEA BRAT #4	SAF-RON GOLD

Source: OIG analysis of NCP Technical Notebook SFT results and ORD's report. Column 1 is an average of two oils using the SFT. Columns 2 and 3 are for one oil using the BFT.

Note: There were differences in testing protocol between the SFT conducted for the schedule and this study; therefore, we limited comparability of information to ranking efficacy test results.

---

[4] Corexit EC9527A was not one of the eight dispersants tested because, as we noted in chapter 1, the standing inventory of EC9527A was depleted and EC9500A became the primary dispersant used during the response. We did not have BFT results for Corexit EC9527A and could not include it in our analysis.

Conclusion

When the Deepwater Horizon oil spill occurred in April 2010, EPA used dispersant efficacy data on the Production Schedule that were based on the SFT. If EPA had updated Subpart J to include the BFT as the standard testing protocol, more reliable efficacy data would have been readily available at the time of the spill.

Recommendation

We recommend that the Assistant Administrator for Solid Waste and Emergency Response:

1. Develop appropriate NCP Subpart J testing revisions, including proceeding with plans in place before the Deepwater Horizon oil spill, to incorporate the most appropriate efficacy testing protocol. Develop an action plan with milestones for these and any other necessary revisions and take steps to propose NCP Subpart J revisions.

Agency Comments and OIG Evaluation

In its response to our official draft report, OSWER generally agreed with recommendation 1. OSWER also provided comments on the report text. OSWER stated that, even with the additional information provided by the BFT, the dispersant used in the Deepwater Horizon oil spill would likely not have changed, and that lessons learned from the spill have informed an ongoing examination of Subpart J. While this may have been the case, we maintain that more reliable data may have been available had OSWER proceeded with its plan to update Subpart J prior to the spill. We revised our report text as appropriate based on OSWER's response. Appendix C includes OSWER's full response, and appendix D includes our evaluation.

Chapter 3
EPA Increased Its Involvement During Deepwater Horizon Oil Spill

We found that responders to the Deepwater Horizon oil spill could have used other dispersants in the response, but not within the window of time afforded by Addendum 2 to the pertinent Joint Directive. We also found that EPA involved senior officials in daily dispersant decisions in addition to the Agency's representative to the RRT. Prior to a spill occurring in deep waters, EPA is one of several agencies responsible for contingency planning, including worst-case discharges, and for listing products on the NCP Product Schedule. During an actual spill response, EPA has responsibilities on the NRT and on RRTs. Section 910 of the NCP discusses the concurrence role for authorization of dispersant use associated with the EPA RRT representative. OSWER said that concurrence authority is not exclusive and does not prohibit involvement of senior management. While we agree that EPA's Administrator retains delegated authority, we found that EPA's involvement of senior Agency officials, in addition to the RRT representative, created confusion on roles and responsibilities. EPA's involvement in dispersant decisions was primarily due to USCG's request given concerns surrounding the use of dispersants and subsea application. We identified two main reasons why EPA involved senior officials during the spill:

- EPA was not prepared for this unprecedented spill, including the volume and duration of dispersant use, and subsea dispersant application.
- EPA and others needed additional clarity on roles and responsibilities for a response to a Spill of National Significance.

Other Dispersants Could Have Been Used but Not in the Time Afforded by the Joint Directive

The first Hotline complaint we received alleged that EPA approved the use of Corexit when other, less harmful substances could have been used. Dispersants EPA lists on the NCP Product Schedule "may be authorized for use" by the designated FOSC. Subpart J of the NCP requires RRTs to address the desirability of using dispersants as a part of their planning activities. Regional and Area Contingency Plans must include, as appropriate, pre-authorization plans that address the specific contexts in which to use such products. The Region 6 RRT granted pre-authorization to the FOSC for dispersant use as defined by the *RRT 6 FOSC Dispersant Pre-approval Guidelines and Checklist*. The plan says, "The only requirement for dispersant product selection is that the dispersant must be included on the NCP Product Schedule and considered appropriate by the FOSC for existing environmental and physical conditions."

As the FOSC, the USCG approved BP's request to use Corexit EC9527A, followed by Corexit EC9500A, in the response. On May 20, 2010, EPA and the USCG issued Addendum 2 to the Joint Directive they had issued to BP. The addendum required BP to identify and use one or more approved dispersants from the Product Schedule that were available in sufficient quantities and were less toxic and as effective as Corexit EC9500A. In addition, Addendum 2 required BP to respond to EPA within 24 hours and use the alternate dispersant identified within 96 hours of the Addendum's issuance and after receiving EPA's approval.

BP responded that no other dispersants that met the acute toxicity and effectiveness criteria in Addendum 2 were available in sufficient quantities to be useful at the time of the spill. According to manufacturers we spoke with, BP contacted a number of them to determine production capacities and inventories available. All manufacturers indicated to BP that they could meet the production requirements but needed 3 to 10 days to ramp up production. BP maintained that Corexit EC9500A remained the best dispersant option. Dissatisfied with BP's response, EPA contacted manufacturers to verify production capacity and conducted its own toxicity testing on eight dispersants.

BP chose the Corexit product as the dispersant to use due to prevalence and national and international stockpiles at the time of the response. In addition, BP's Gulf of Mexico Regional Oil Spill Plan listed the Corexit dispersants in over 99 percent of dispersants inventoried. EPA and the USCG interviewees said Corexit has been tested many times, is well known, and responders are comfortable with using it in a spill response.

EPA and the USCG issued Addendum 2 due to the volume of dispersants used and because EPA said it received public concerns to use a less toxic dispersant. In testimony before the House Energy and Commerce Subcommittee on Energy and the Environment, Administrator Lisa P. Jackson said EPA will continue to push BP to switch to less toxic alternatives due to the volumes of the dispersants being used and the lengthening period of this crisis. EPA staff said the Agency conducted its own toxicity testing on available dispersants to ensure that it based decisions about ongoing dispersant use on the best available science. EPA staff said its tests were consistent with those required by Subpart J but were conducted by one laboratory for comparability of results. EPA said it did this rather than rely solely on test data provided by the Product Schedule with test results conducted at different times by different laboratories. Additionally, EPA staff said its tests used Louisiana Sweet Crude Oil rather than #2 Fuel Oil (stipulated in the NCP) to increase applicability of results to the Gulf situation. Finally, OEM's Regulation and Policy Development Director said its tests also addressed BP's potential endocrine disruptor concern.

During the spill, EPA used staff resources to obtain more information than was available on the NCP Product Schedule. EPA's toxicity testing results, issued on

June 30, 2010, verified that results were consistent with the schedule, and indicated that none of the eight dispersants tested displayed biologically significant endocrine disrupting activity. EPA's testing results did not affect which dispersant responders used; Corexit was the only dispersant used in the response. Responders could have used other dispersants, but manufacturers would have needed more time to ramp up their production than the window of time afforded by Addendum 2. Three of the five dispersant manufacturers contacted believed they wasted their time in responding to various requests for information, that responders never really considered their products, and that responders did not capture their production capabilities. OSWER said it was not able to obtain consistent information on production capacities from some manufacturers, and that the Agency worked during the spill to be as transparent and open as possible with manufacturers.

EPA Was Not Prepared for the Unprecedented Volume and Duration of Dispersant Use and Subsea Application

Contingency plans we reviewed were out of date at the time of the Deepwater Horizon oil spill and were not updated to reflect deepwater drilling trends, lessons learned from a 2002 Spill of National Significance exercise, and past major oil spills. The OPA improved the nation's ability to prevent and respond to oil spills and provided requirements for contingency planning. The NCP further outlines these requirements and states that Contingency Plans shall be adequate to remove a worst-case discharge and mitigate or prevent a substantial threat of such a discharge. However, there is no specific requirement to update contingency plans under the NCP or OPA. Improved contingency planning using available information could have better prepared EPA to support USCG's response to the spill.

Various documents address contingency planning:

- OPA established provisions that expanded the federal government's responsibility and resources to respond to oil spills. OPA provided new requirements for contingency planning by both government and industry.
- The NCP outlines requirements for Regional and Area Contingency Plans:
  - Subpart C requires each designated area to develop a plan adequate to remove a worst-case discharge and to mitigate or prevent a substantial threat of such a discharge.
  - Subpart J states that RRTs and Area Committees should address the desirability of using various products on the NCP Product Schedule based on certain environmental conditions. Plans should include applicable pre-authorization plans that address the specific contexts in which to use such products.
- The Region 6 RRT Regional Integrated Contingency Plan calls for continuous reviews on the effectiveness and integration of all plans based on actual response experiences, exercises, and other relevant information (including the spill history of an area) that will lead to enhanced plans.

Region 6 RRT contingency plans were outdated at the time of the Deepwater Horizon oil spill. The Region 6 RRT completed an interim update to non-dispersant sections in the Regional Integrated Contingency Plan on May 20, 2010, subsequent to the explosion that caused the Deepwater Horizon oil spill. The *RRT-6 FOSC Dispersant Pre-approval Guidelines and Checklist* was last updated in 2001. One EPA official described plan revisions as a very detailed and complicated process, but said a catastrophic event would trigger updates to contingency plans. Plans were not updated to address the following events:

- A dramatic expansion of deepwater drilling in the Gulf of Mexico. Oil production in the Gulf grew from 275 million barrels in 1990, where 4.4 percent came from deepwater wells, to 567 million barrels in 2009, where deepwater wells yielded more than 80 percent of the total. In addition, from 2001 to 2004, 11 major oil fields were discovered in water depths of 7,000 feet or more. Figure 2 shows the increase in water depth of wells drilled in the Gulf from 1940 to 2010.

- Lessons learned from a Gulf of Mexico Spill of National Significance exercise in 2002 stating that pre-authorization plans should address potential shortfalls of dispersant supplies and equipment. The lessons learned document assigned EPA and the USCG as the steward agencies, yet plans were not updated to address potential dispersant shortfalls. OSWER said that dispersants were not used in this exercise but agreed that pre-authorization plans should address potential shortfalls of dispersant supplies and equipment.

- Hurricanes Katrina and Rita in 2004 and 2005, which collectively destroyed 113 oil platforms, 70 vessels, and nearly 130 oil and natural gas pipelines, and ravaged the Gulf Coast with major impacts to offshore infrastructure and operations.

Figure 2: Depth of wells in the Gulf of Mexico, 1940 to 2010

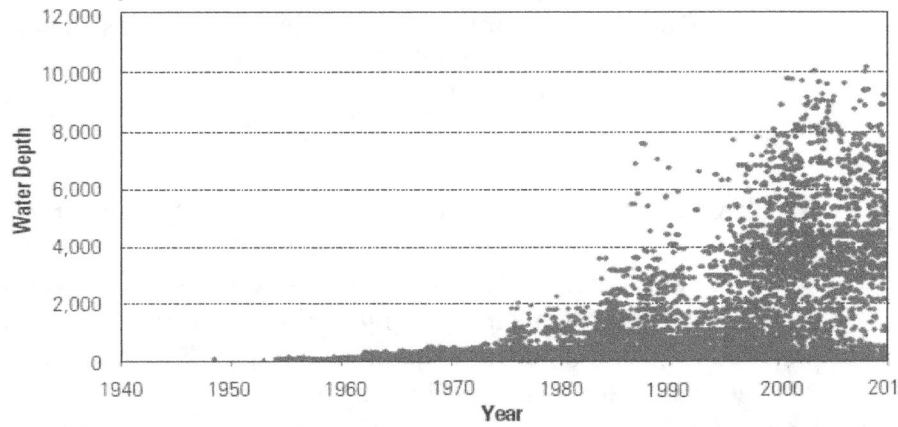

Source: National Commission on the BP Deepwater Horizon Oil Spill and Offshore Drilling, Final Report (January 2011), based on data from the Bureau of Ocean Energy Management, Regulation, and Enforcement within the Department of the Interior.

Further, contingency plans were not updated based on other historical spills. The 2010 Region 6 RRT Regional Integrated Contingency Plan defines a major discharge as greater than 100,000 gallons in coastal waters. The Ixtoc I spill in the Gulf of Mexico in 1979 released 3.3 million barrels of oil and lasted over 10 months. Between 1 million and 2.5 million gallons of mostly Corexit

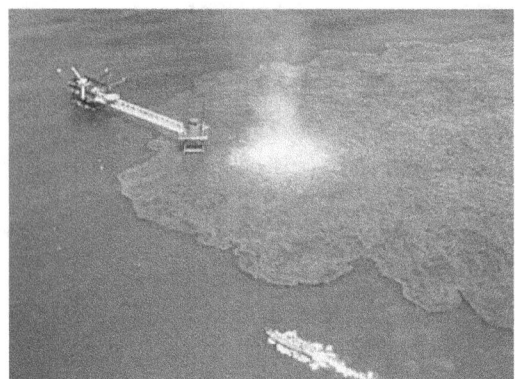

dispersant products were applied. OSWER said lessons from this 1979 spill were available before the contingency plan was drafted. However, we found that knowledge gained from this spill was not considered by the Region 6 RRT when drafting its Regional Integrated Contingency Plan to better address worst-case discharges and spill duration. In addition, ORD's Assistant Administrator said ORD would have liked to have more data and insight from the Ixtoc I spill to build into decisionmaking for future spills.

The Ixtoc oil spill. (National Oceanic and Atmospheric Administration photo)

During the Deepwater Horizon oil spill, a number of concerns were not addressed in contingency plans, especially with regard to dispersants. For example, one EPA director described the novel approach of applying dispersants subsurface as "somewhat trial and error." Concerns included questions on the potential impact of the volume of dispersants applied, effectiveness of dispersants at such low temperatures, oil weathering as it rose to the surface, and environmental effects on the deep sea. The Region 6 RRT Regional Integrated Contingency Plan itself lists one of the disadvantages of dispersants as "lots of unknowns."

The Region 6 RRT did not update its plans because there is no requirement to do so. Even though the Region 6 RRT Regional Integrated Contingency Plan calls for the RRT to continuously review the effectiveness of plans, the NCP and OPA do not require plans to be reviewed and updated. Response plans contained boilerplate language taken from the NCP with slight variation based on local geography. For example, the section on Chemical Countermeasures in the Region 6 RRT Regional Integrated Contingency Plan essentially repeats the information in Subpart J of the NCP. The plan does not address Region 6 RRT-specific issues such as logistical boundaries where dispersants may not be used or discussion of the pre-authorization plan.

An EPA Region 6 division director said he did not believe EPA could have anticipated a spill of this magnitude, and OSWER said that the dispersant pre-approval plan was not anticipated for long-term use. However, more detailed and updated contingency planning using available information could have better prepared EPA and others to respond to the spill. Future planning should consider the Deepwater Horizon scenario and address worst-case discharges, lessons learned from Spill of National Significance exercises, and industry trends. OEM staff said the RRT is working to revisit the conditions associated with dispersants under the pre-authorization plans. Additionally, on November 2, 2010, OSWER's Assistant Administrator provided interim actions to RRTs to address issues raised during the Deepwater Horizon oil spill. The interim actions call for Area and Regional Contingency Plans to consider various conditions and limitations to dispersants. The interim actions said plans should consider site-specific and oil-specific rationale for environmental trade-offs and favorable dispersant use conditions, as well as a process for longer-term responses and the need for monitoring information to reassess dispersant use.

Additional Clarity Needed on Roles and Responsibilities for Responses to Spills of National Significance

Additional guidance is needed on the roles and responsibilities for responding to a Spill of National Significance. As the first Spill of National Significance in the United States, and due to the unprecedented nature of the spill, EPA increased its involvement during the Deepwater Horizon response. EPA's involvement was primarily due to USCG's request given concerns surrounding the use of dispersants and subsea application. EPA was involved and concurred with the decision to use dispersants subsurface, issued a Joint Directive and Addenda with the USCG to BP, and became involved in daily operational dispersant decisions. The NCP and the National Response Framework allow the response structure to adjust to include senior Agency officials, especially when responding to a Spill of National Significance. However, the NCP does not provide guidance on the roles and responsibilities of the National Incident Commander and other high-level officials. As a result, involvement of senior EPA officials created confusion as to who in EPA made dispersant decisions.

Under the NCP, for spills occurring in coastal zones, EPA is responsible for planning prior to a spill and supporting the USCG during a response. The NCP states that for a Spill of National Significance in the coastal zone, the USCG may name a National Incident Commander who assumes the role of the OSC in communicating with affected parties and coordinating resources at the national level. The NCP further states that coordination will involve the NRT, RRTs, and others as appropriate. However, the NCP does not address how high-level officials other than the National Incident Commander can and should participate in such a response.

Responders encountered a number of unique circumstances in the Deepwater Horizon oil spill, such as the spill lasting 87 days and using close to 2 million gallons of dispersants. Through its role as NRT chair, EPA became involved in the decision to use dispersants subsurface at the request of the USCG FOSC. Subsurface application was a novel approach to oil spill mitigation, and there was limited knowledge on the effects of applying dispersants a mile below the surface. EPA and the USCG issued a Joint Directive and Addendum 1 to BP outlining a subsurface dispersant monitoring plan. EPA had never issued a joint directive with the USCG before, and this action allowed the Agency to become more involved in the spill response, as EPA and the USCG held BP accountable for following the Directive.

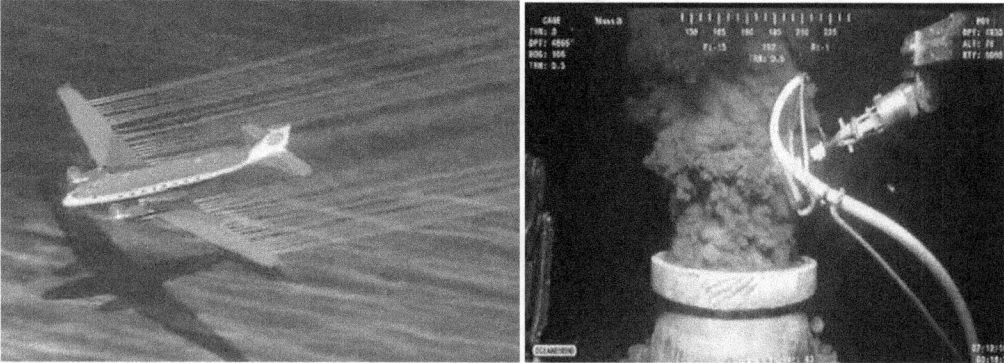

From left: An example of surface dispersant application (USCG photo); an example of a subsurface dispersant application (image taken from Macondo video feed; photograph republished from MSNBC/AP with permission from BP).

On May 26, 2010, EPA and the USCG issued Addendum 3 to the Directive and required BP to limit the use of dispersants subsurface to 15,000 gallons per day and eliminate surface application except when granted exemption. It was unclear in our review what scientific basis responders used to set the 15,000-gallon limit. The Addendum sought to limit dispersant use and require more documentation because of concerns about ongoing dispersant applications in such large volumes. Given unknowns on the long-term health and environmental effects of dispersants, EPA wanted to use the least amount possible to be effective. Because of the Deepwater Horizon oil spill, Congress appropriated $2.0 million to EPA to support research on the short- and long-term environmental and public health implications associated with the spill and surface/subsurface dispersant applications. ORD plans to further its research efforts to include innovative and expansive approaches to spill remediation.

Rather than EPA's involvement occurring though the RRT and NRT as would happen in a typical response under the NCP, senior EPA officials became involved in daily surface dispersant decisions. The Agency was concerned about the precedent-setting amount of dispersants used and the number of exemptions the USCG granted with minimal justification. On June 9, 2010, EPA developed a hierarchy of decisionmaking intended to give staff-level EPA RRT representatives on the ground some role in daily decisionmaking on surface exemptions. However, internal communications indicated that senior Agency officials made decisions on surface applications. Key staff in Region 6, including EPA's representative to the Region 6 RRT and staff involved in the response, said they did not have the decisionmaking authority for the Agency to approve dispersant applications. However, our review showed they were involved in gathering information for decisionmaking by senior EPA officials. One Region 6 response official described the process as "very political" and said "operational control was taken away from the region." As a result, EPA's involvement of senior officials in daily surface application decisions created confusion as to who in the Agency made decisions. In its response to our draft report, OSWER said that the RRT representative was heavily involved in the decisionmaking process, and that the decisionmaking process included RRT and NRT members. OSWER also said that senior Agency officials in Area Command, in consultation with EPA's representatives in the Incident Command, gave concurrence to the FOSC.

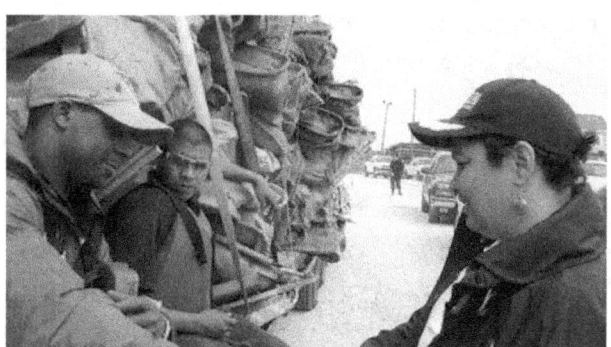

EPA Administrator Jackson during one Gulf trip.
(Photo from www.RestoreTheGulf.gov).

EPA's Administrator increased her involvement, as well as that of other senior Agency officials, due to the novel approach of applying dispersants subsurface, the size and nature of the spill, the volume of dispersants used, and political interest.[5] In our interview with Administrator Jackson, she said, "As good as our field staff is, I was not going to have the response progress without a senior set of eyes . . . especially when you have the White House involved. . . . " Additionally, in her testimony on July 15, 2010, the Administrator said, "I think a unified command makes sense for smaller spills, but on something like this, there needs to be additional clarity."

The concurrence process in place for surface dispersant application created delays as EPA established a process requiring decisions be elevated to the OSWER Assistant Administrator and, at times, to the Administrator. EPA senior officials believe their involvement in the decision to apply dispersants subsurface reduced the total amount of dispersants applied overall (subsurface and surface). EPA officials also believe subsurface dispersant application was effective. In its response to our draft report, OSWER said that all decisions regarding dispersants and involving senior officials were clearly and appropriately vetted through the NRT and the RRT, and that EPA acted consistent with the NCP in concurring on the USCG FOSC's decisions. However, as the President's Commission Report noted, due to insufficient guidance on roles and responsibilities for a Spill of National Significance, additional protocol is needed that accounts for participation by high-level officials. OSWER agrees with the need for additional clarity on roles and responsibilities, as well as coordination and communication, for responding to a Spill of National Significance.

Conclusion

Due to concerns surrounding the unprecedented volume and duration of dispersant use and subsea application, EPA involved senior officials in addition to the RRT representative. While Subpart J of the NCP discusses the RRT

---

[5] A number of EPA officials testified before Congress. Throughout the spill and after the well was capped, the EPA Administrator testified four times, the Deputy Administrator testified once, and ORD officials testified four times. In addition, EPA participated in hearings before the National Commission on the BP Deepwater Horizon Oil Spill. Political officials asked EPA questions on its roles and responsibilities in an oil spill response and the health and environmental effects of dispersants.

representatives' concurrence role for dispersant use, it does not preclude the involvement of senior officials. However, EPA's involvement of senior Agency officials in dispersant decisions created confusion within and outside the Agency. Additionally, EPA did not update plans and was not prepared for a spill of this magnitude, including the subsea use of dispersants. EPA could better respond to future significant spills by enhancing planning efforts to address unknowns encountered in the Deepwater Horizon response and by clarifying roles and responsibilities of senior Agency officials.

Recommendations

We recommend that the Assistant Administrator for Solid Waste and Emergency Response:

2. Have the OEM Director work through the office's NRT capacity to establish a policy that calls for periodic reviews and updates to contingency plans, after considering lessons learned from major national and international oil spills, and/or based on area trends in oil drilling.

3. Modify the NCP Product Schedule and contingency plans to include additional information (such as testing on crude oil, subsurface dispersants application, volume and duration limits, etc.) learned from the Deepwater Horizon oil spill response and use such information to revise and update Area and Regional Contingency Plans.

4. Develop policies/procedures for subsurface dispersant application and modify pre-authorization plans to address subsurface use.

5. Develop guidance and training for a Spill of National Significance that clarifies roles and responsibilities for high-level Agency officials. Review this response and the NCP and work with federal partners to address lessons learned and include detail on how to respond to a Spill of National Significance.

6. Review and analyze NCP Subpart J toxicity testing protocols to ensure that emergency responders have the information necessary for appropriate subsurface dispersant use for future oil spills.

7. As part of the action to review NCP Subpart J requirements, address the need to capture and maintain dispersant manufacturer production capacities, equipment requirements, and other necessary information to better prepare for future oil spills. Make this information widely available to the response community.

We recommend that the Assistant Administrator for Research and Development:

8. Develop a research plan to address gaps on long-term health and environmental effects of dispersants.

Agency Comments and OIG Evaluation

In ORD's response to our draft report, ORD agreed with recommendation 8. ORD indicated that it has already taken steps to address this recommendation, such as developing a longer-term strategy to address gaps specifically related to the health and environmental effects of dispersants and other oil-spill-related research needs. We concur with ORD's planned actions. We will make final determinations on these actions once we review ORD's corrective action plan and milestone dates to address our recommendation, and this recommendation is unresolved with resolution efforts in progress. Appendix E contains ORD's response.

OSWER generally agreed with our recommendations. OSWER's response included comments on the text in chapter 3, most notably on the unprecedented nature of the Deepwater Horizon oil spill. We agree with OSWER on the magnitude of the spill, and we did not intend to imply that EPA's support to the USCG was inadequate or that decisions were inappropriate. We believe that our findings and corresponding recommendations align with the fact that this event was unprecedented, and that EPA should take action to address lessons learned. We discussed OSWER's response and our disposition in two meetings wherein we focused on EPA's role under the NCP. OSWER and EPA's Office of General Counsel provided us the following information, which we summarized in chapter 1:

> The Deepwater Horizon Oil Spill was declared a Spill of National Significance. When there is a Spill of National Significance, the FOSC assigned by the USCG for a coastal spill can appoint a National Incident Commander. Under 40 CFR 300.323(c) of the NCP, the National Incident Commander has the authority to coordinate federal, State, local, or national resources for the response. It is our understanding that the National Incident Commander called upon the EPA Administrator for involvement in various response actions, including the use of dispersants.
>
> The NCP also provides for NRT involvement in a response, particularly in novel or significant situations. Please see 40 CFR 300.110.
>
> While 40 CFR 300.910 discusses the concurrence role for authorization of dispersant use associated with the EPA RRT representative, that concurrence authority is not exclusive and does

not prohibit the involvement of senior management. The authority, jurisdiction, and implementation provisions in the NCP flow from Section 311 of the Clean Water Act and are reflected in Executive Order 12777. All authorities under CWA 311 are delegated either directly to the Administrator by Congress, or by Executive Order 12777 from the President to the Administrator. While the Administrator's authority may be further delegated through senior management on down to the RRT representative, the Administrator (and other delegatees) retain the authority to act. The mere delegation of authority does not prohibit the delegator from exercising said authority.

OSWER agreed with recommendations 2, 3, 4, and 6, and stated that work is already underway to address most of the recommendations. We will make final determinations on these actions once we review OSWER's corrective action plan and milestone dates to address our recommendations, and these recommendations are unresolved with resolution efforts in progress. OSWER suggested the following revision to recommendation 5: "Develop training for a Spill of National Significance event that clarifies roles and responsibilities for high-level Agency officials. Review the response and work with federal partners to address lessons learned." We do not entirely agree with this revision because training alone may not fully address lessons learned from the response. We believe that, in addition to training, EPA should develop guidance based on lessons learned and be open to considering any necessary revisions to the NCP. We revised recommendation 5 to include some of OSWER's suggested language. For recommendation 7, OSWER said that the proposed rule on Subpart J revisions may ask for comment on the manufacturer being responsible for tracking production capacities. We recognize this and adjusted our recommendation. Appendix C includes OSWER's full response, and appendix D includes our evaluation of that response.

Status of Recommendations and Potential Monetary Benefits

		RECOMMENDATIONS				POTENTIAL MONETARY BENEFITS (in $000s)	
Rec. No.	Page No.	Subject	Status[1]	Action Official	Planned Completion Date	Claimed Amount	Agreed To Amount
1	11	Develop appropriate NCP Subpart J testing revisions, including proceeding with plans in place before the Deepwater Horizon oil spill, to incorporate the most appropriate efficacy testing protocol. Develop an action plan with milestones for these and any other necessary revisions and take steps to propose NCP Subpart J revisions.	U	Assistant Administrator for Solid Waste and Emergency Response			
2	20	Have the OEM Director work through the office's NRT capacity to establish a policy that calls for periodic reviews and updates to contingency plans, after considering lessons learned from major national and international oil spills, and/or based on area trends in oil drilling.	U	Assistant Administrator for Solid Waste and Emergency Response			
3	20	Modify the NCP Product Schedule and contingency plans to include additional information (such as testing on crude oil, subsurface dispersants application, volume and duration limits, etc.) learned from the Deepwater Horizon oil spill response and use such information to revise and update Area and Regional Contingency Plans.	U	Assistant Administrator for Solid Waste and Emergency Response			
4	20	Develop policies/procedures for subsurface dispersant application and modify pre-authorization plans to address subsurface use.	U	Assistant Administrator for Solid Waste and Emergency Response			
5	20	Develop guidance and training for a Spill of National Significance that clarifies roles and responsibilities for high-level Agency officials. Review this response and the NCP and work with federal partners to address lessons learned and include detail on how to respond to a Spill of National Significance.	U	Assistant Administrator for Solid Waste and Emergency Response			
6	20	Review and analyze NCP Subpart J toxicity testing protocols to ensure that emergency responders have the information necessary for appropriate subsurface dispersant use for future oil spills.	U	Assistant Administrator for Solid Waste and Emergency Response			
7	20	As part of the action to review NCP Subpart J requirements, address the need to capture and maintain dispersant manufacturer production capacities, equipment requirements, and other necessary information to better prepare for future oil spills. Make this information widely available to the response community.	U	Assistant Administrator for Solid Waste and Emergency Response			
8	21	Develop a research plan to address gaps on long-term health and environmental effects of dispersants.	U	Assistant Administrator for Research and Development			

[1] O = recommendation is open with agreed-to corrective actions pending
C = recommendation is closed with all agreed-to actions completed
U = recommendation is unresolved with resolution efforts in progress

Details on Scope and Methodology

We conducted our review to address two Hotline complaints on use of dispersants in the Deepwater Horizon oil spill. We sought to determine what steps EPA took to analyze the dispersant Corexit to include it on the NCP Product Schedule, as well as EPA's role in the decision to use Corexit over other dispersants. To address both objectives, we reviewed and summarized relevant laws, regulations, and guidance on oil spill response, including the NCP, OPA, CWA, and Executive Order 12777. We reviewed activities by several EPA offices, including OSWER, OEM, ORD, Region 6, and the Administrator's office. We also interviewed key USCG officials given that the USCG served as the lead response agency.

To address our first objective we:

- Analyzed the NCP Product Schedule and reviewed information submitted by the manufacturer of Corexit to get listed on the schedule.
- Interviewed current and former Product Schedule Managers in OEM to determine the process of including a product on the Product Schedule.
- Interviewed an EPA contractor about its role supporting OEM in reviewing submissions for the NCP Product Schedule, including the contractor's analysis of manufacturer-submitted requirements and staff qualifications.
- Reviewed proposed revisions EPA planned for Subpart J of the NCP before the Deepwater Horizon oil spill occurred and met with OSWER and OEM officials to discuss necessary revisions to Subpart J as a result of the spill.
- Interviewed former OEM Regulation and Policy Development Division Directors to understand why revisions to Subpart J of the NCP were not finalized before the Deepwater Horizon spill.
- Interviewed an ORD dispersant expert to gain an understanding of dispersants and efficacy testing protocols, including the SFT and BFT.

To address our second objective we:

- Documented the timeline of events of the Deepwater Horizon oil spill to understand the sequence of events and highlight EPA's activities.
- Reviewed contingency plans from the Region 6 RRT as well as BP's *Gulf of Mexico Regional Oil Spill Response Plan* to understand the level of preparation plans provided during the response as well as the organizational structure underlying the response.
- Reviewed congressional testimony from EPA's Administrator, Deputy Administrator, Assistant Administrator for ORD, and an ORD Division Director.
- To understand EPA's involvement throughout the response, including decision making on dispersants, interviewed:
  - The Administrator
  - Deputy Administrator
  - Assistant Administrators for OSWER and ORD

- o Acting Director and other key staff within OEM
- o The Director of the Superfund Division and key staff in Region 6, including EPA's representative to the Region 6 RRT and staff involved in the response.
- To understand the role of EPA versus that of the USCG, interviewed the Admiral appointed as National Incident Commander, FOSCs who served during the 87-day response, and USCG's deputy area commander and representative to the Region 6 RRT. Also, reviewed e-mails and other documentation provided by the USCG.
- Reviewed documentation, meeting notes, and e-mails from Region 6, OSWER, and ORD, including the Joint Directive and Addenda from EPA and the USCG, to understand the flow of communication regarding the surface and subsurface use of dispersants.
- Attended a National Science Foundation Dispersant Workshop and a Clean Gulf Conference to gain insight into the oil spill response industry and the role that dispersants have during a response.
- Conducted research on dispersants, including dispersant testing protocols and stockpiles.
- Interviewed dispersant manufacturers to determine availability and production capacity of their products and whether responders considered their products during the spill.

In May 2010, President Obama established the National Commission on the BP Deepwater Horizon Oil Spill and Offshore Drilling through Executive Order 13543. The commission examined the relevant facts and circumstances concerning the root causes of the Deepwater Horizon explosion, fire, and spill and options to mitigate the impact of future spills. We reviewed staff working papers and the final report, issued to the President in January 2011, to assess the Commission's review and relevance on our two objectives.

The OIG Office of Counsel addressed components of the Hotline complaint alleging that the EPA Administrator and employees committed perjury. Office of Counsel reviewed testimony by EPA senior officials to determine whether evidence demonstrated that perjury existed. Appendix B summarizes Office of Counsel's perjury review results.

Allegation of Perjury by Senior EPA Officials in Congressional Testimony

We received a Hotline complaint on July 25, 2010, asserting, among other matters, that EPA was covering up the effects of the Corexit dispersant. The Hotline referred to claims by an EPA employee that Administrator Jackson perjured herself in testimony before Senator Mikulski on July 15, 2010, by making false statements that Gulf air and water are safe. Our Office of Counsel reviewed allegations concerning perjury and did not address the cover-up allegation. In its response to our draft report, the Agency denied any cover-up and said that it took aggressive steps to affirmatively disclose data regarding dispersant use. We noted the Agency's response on this point in chapter 1 of our report under "Noteworthy Achievements."

Even though the perjury allegation only identified the testimony given by the Administrator on July 15, 2010, our Office of Counsel reviewed nine sworn statements (including that given by the Administrator on July 15, 2010), and related responses to "Questions for the Record," provided by senior EPA officials to Congress during the response. To determine whether any such evidence of perjury existed, our Office of Counsel relied on the legal definition of perjury and the following three required elements of a perjury offense:

1. The first element is that the party must be under oath during their testimony, declaration, or certification.
2. The second element is that the party must have made a false statement.
3. The third element is proof of specific intent, that is, that the party made the false statement with knowledge of its falsity, rather than because of confusion, mistake or faulty memory. The false statement must be material to the proceedings. A false statement is material if it has "a natural tendency to influence, or is capable of influencing, the decision of the decision-making body to which it was addressed."

The review did not find evidence supporting the elements of perjury. As none of the testimony reviewed demonstrated any evidence that tended to indicate that senior EPA officials committed perjury, the OIG did not make any recommendations to EPA on allegations of perjury raised in the Hotline complaint.

OSWER's Response to Draft Report

June 30, 2011

MEMORANDUM

SUBJECT: Environmental Protection Agency's (EPA) Response to OIG's Draft Report:
                      *"Revisions Needed to National Contingency Plan Based on Deepwater Horizon
                      Oil Spill,"* Project No. OA-FY10-0221

FROM   Mathy Stanislaus
                      Assistant Administrator

TO: Melissa M. Heist
                      Assistant Inspector General for Audit

We appreciate the opportunity to comment on the Office of Inspector General (OIG) draft audit
report: *"Revisions Needed to National Contingency Plan Based on Deepwater Horizon Oil Spill"*
(Project No. OA-FY10-0221), dated May 24, 2011.

The Deepwater Horizon (DWH) Oil Spill was an unprecedented event requiring an extraordinary
response. Throughout the course of the spill and for a time following the capping of the well,
EPA collected, analyzed and posted data on the Agency's website for over 5,000 air, waste,
sediment, and water samples; developed and implemented policies associated with the
unanticipated use of dispersants necessitated by this event; conducted scientific testing in
expedient timeframes; and demonstrated proactive efforts to improve operations. Although the
report recognizes many of the Agency's accomplishments and we generally agree with the
recommendations, there are portions requiring clarification, and we modified the fifth and
seventh recommendations.

The report does not accurately delineate the roles of EPA and the U.S. Coast Guard (USCG) in
the DWH response. Under the National Contingency Plan (NCP), the USCG is the lead agency
in response to **coastal** oil spills. EPA is the lead agency in response to inland oil spills. In this
event, EPA supported the USCG and worked with federal partners to ensure timely and
responsible decisions. In this regard, the statement that "EPA was not prepared for quantity and
duration of dispersant use" (pp 11 and 13) should be clarified to avoid the implication that the
support EPA provided to the USCG was inadequate. EPA acknowledges that the quantity and
duration of dispersant use were unprecedented during the DWH Spill of National Significance
(SONS) event.

EPA mobilized quickly and efficiently in support of the federal spill response. Numerous
activities demonstrate EPA's contributions, including deployment of personnel and equipment
into the field, enhanced monitoring activities, daily public data posting, collaboration and
cooperation with federal partners, involvement and expertise of EPA's research community to

support decision making with sound science, development of waste management strategies and incorporation of environmental justice concerns into any and all decision-making. Throughout the course of the spill, EPA conducted this work at the highest level of scientific integrity, while adapting and responding rapidly to ever-changing conditions and challenges of a crisis.

Our specific comments (provided in the Attachment) address concerns that require attention and consideration. Should you have any questions, please contact Dana Tulis in the Office of Emergency Management at (202) 564-8600. We appreciate your efforts and your incorporation of our comments as you develop the final report.

This transmittal covers responses to recommendations regarding OSWER. Assistant Administrator Paul Anastas has indicated that he will respond separately regarding recommendations applicable to ORD.

Attachment

cc: Paul Anastas

ATTACHMENT

Specific comments are detailed below by section and chapter:

"At a Glance"

1. *"… EPA did not proceed with rulemaking before the Deepwater Horizon oil spill occurred because of competing priorities and changes in management. If EPA had updated Subpart J, more reliable efficacy data could have been readily available during the oil spill."*   Although this is true, only three of the eight dispersant products tested by EPA for effectiveness using the preferred Baffled Flask Test would pass proposed efficacy criteria. One of the three is the dispersant used in the spill. Consequently, even with this additional information, the dispersant used in this spill would likely not have changed. Separately, the lessons learned from DWH have informed an on-going examination of Subpart J.

2. *"EPA increased its involvement because (a) it was not prepared for the amount of the dispersant use, and (b) additional clarity was needed on roles and responsibilities in responding to a Spill of National Significance. EPA's increased involvement created confusion as to who at EPA led response efforts for dispersant use."*   EPA increased its involvement not because it wasn't prepared for the amount of dispersant use but because the amount of dispersant use was unprecedented. EPA has decision-making authority under Subpart J of the NCP. The EPA representative to the Regional Response Team (RRT) must concur on any pre-authorization for the use of chemical agents (such as dispersants, surface washing agents, surface collecting agents, bioremediation agents, and miscellaneous oil spill agents) for any oil spill. The EPA representative to the RRT must also concur on the use of chemical agents for spill situations not addressed by pre-

authorization plans. During the Deepwater Horizon spill, EPA was consulted and responded in an expeditious manner.

Chapter 1

1. Page 2, *"For a Spill of National Significance, Subpart D of the NCP states that USCG [United States Coast Guard] and EPA can name a National Incident Commander to assume the role of OSC for spills occurring in coastal and inland zones, respectively."* The statement does not fully reflect 40CFR300.323. The USCG appoints the FOSC in the coastal zone and EPA appoints the FOSC in the inland zone. The "National Incident Commander" title is used in 40CFR300.323 only for the coastal zone.

2. Page 4, *"The spill lasted 87 days and spilled an estimated 4.9 million barrels of oil, making it the largest marine oil spill in U.S. history."* OIG should note that investigation into the number of barrels spilled is ongoing.

Chapter 2

1. Page 1, *"The BFT [Baffled Flask Test] has proved more reproducible, and if EPA had updated Subpart J to include it as the standard testing protocol, more reliable efficacy data would have been readily available at the time of the Deepwater Horizon oil spill."* As noted above, it is true more reliable efficacy data would have been available at the time of the spill. But test results shows that this data may not have made any difference in the dispersant used.

2. Table 2, *"Dispersant Efficacy Ranking Using SFT [Swirling Flask Test] and BFT [Baffled Flask Test]"* may be misleading. The efficacy test data in Column 1 is an average of two oils using the SFT while the data in Columns 2 and 3 is for only one oil using the BFT. The underlying data confirms that the dispersant used compares well with all those available at the time of the spill.

Chapter 3

1. Page 1, *"We found that responders to the Deepwater Horizon oil spill could have used other dispersants in the response, but not within the window of time afforded by Addendum 2 to the pertinent Joint Directive. Further, we found that EPA increased its involvement in the Deepwater Horizon oil spill response beyond the role envisioned for the Agency in the NCP for deep water spills, due primarily to USCG's request given concerns surrounding the use of dispersants and subsea application."* Choice of dispersants was initially vested in the USCG FOSC. In exercising its concurrence via the Joint Directive, EPA reviewed available information and required additional toxicity testing. EPA increased its involvement given the concerns surrounding the use of dispersants but its role was entirely consistent with the NCP. Prior to the Deepwater Horizon oil spill the US had never used dispersant subsea or in such quantities. Finally, as noted above, the EPA representative to the RRT must concur on any pre-authorization

for the use of chemical agents on any oil spill or on the use of chemical agents for spill situations not addressed by pre-authorization plans.

> See Appendix D, Note 1, for OIG Response.

2. Page 11, *'EPA was not prepared for the amount and length of dispersant use."* The magnitudes of oil spilled and dispersant used were unprecedented. However, this should not imply that EPA's support was inadequate.

3. Page 12, *"Three of the five dispersant manufacturers contacted believed they wasted their time in responding to various requests for information, that responders never really considered their products, and that responders did not capture their production capabilities."* EPA is sympathetic with the manufacturer's concerns. At the same time, as noted above, USCG had the lead for dispersant choice. EPA worked during the spill to be as transparent and open as possible regarding the situation with manufacturers under unusual circumstances and the challenges associated with potentially interrupting the spill response to change products along with whether sufficient quantity could be provided. EPA was not able to obtain consistent information regarding production capacities from some of the manufacturers.

4. Page 13, *"Improved contingency planning using available information could have better prepared EPA to support USCG's response to the spill."* As previously stated, the Deepwater Horizon Oil Spill was an unprecedented event. However, this should not imply that EPA's support to the USCG was inadequate.

5. Page 14, *"Lessons learned from Spill of National Significance exercises in 2002 stating that pre-authorization plans should address potential shortfalls of dispersant supplies and equipment. Hurricanes Katrina and Rita in 2004 and 2005, which collectively destroyed 113 oil platforms, 70 vessels, and nearly 130 oil and natural gas pipelines, and ravaged the Gulf Coast with major impacts to offshore infrastructure and operations."* These statements need clarification. They seem to suggest that dispersants were involved in the exercises and hurricane responses from which EPA could have learned and been better prepared. This is not the case. Although it is true pre-authorization plans should address shortfalls of dispersant supplies and equipment, the exercises and hurricanes did not involve or contemplate the use of dispersants to the extent as in the BP Spill. Note that EPA and USCG did update the area contingency plan (ACP) in spring of 2010. This update was completed in the spring of 2010 despite the responses to Hurricanes Katrina, Rita, Gustav, and Ike.

> See Appendix D, Note 2, for OIG Response.

6. Page 14, *"The Ixtoc I spill in the Gulf of Mexico in 1979 released 3.3 million barrels of oil and lasted over 10 months. The Region 6 RRT could have used knowledge gained from this spill to update its Regional Integrated Contingency Plan to better address worse-case discharges and spill duration."* The Ixtoc Oil Spill in 1979 occurred before OPA existed and before the ACP was developed. Thus, its lessons were available before

the ACP was drafted and we question the record support for the conclusion that the ACP needed updating to reflect it.

> See Appendix D, Note 3, for OIG Response.

7. Page 15, *"An EPA Region 6 Division Director said he did not believe EPA could have anticipated a spill of this magnitude. However, more detailed and updated contingency planning using available information could have better prepared EPA and others to respond to the spill. Future planning should consider the Deepwater Horizon scenario and address worst case discharges, lessons learned from Spill of National Significance exercises, and industry trends."* In context, it seems the Region 6 Division Director was speaking directly to the use of dispersants under the pre-approval plan and the inability of the USCG and the RP to control the release. EPA fulfilled its obligations as a co-chair of the Regional Response Team (RRT), and exercised its concurrence on the use of a dispersant based on the dispersants available. The dispersant pre-approval plan was not anticipated for long-term use, rather pre-approval was developed to assure that the FOSC and/or the RP has appropriate tools for the immediate response to a spill. Because of this, EPA increased its involvement in surface dispersant decisions during the Deepwater Horizon oil spill and instituted procedures to monitor for effects associated with the sub-surface application of dispersants. Region 6 is working within the Region 6 RRT to revisit the conditions associated with dispersant use under the Pre-Authorization Plan.

8. Page 16, *"...the NCP does not provide guidance on the roles and responsibilities of the National Incident Commander and other high-level officials. As a result, involvement by senior EPA officials created confusion as to who made dispersant decisions."* All decisions regarding dispersants and involving senior officials were clearly and appropriately vetted thru the National Response Team (NRT) as well as the RRT.

9. Page 16 *Under the NCP, for spills occurring in coastal zones, EPA is not given any decision-making authority, but EPA is responsible for planning prior to a spill and supporting the USCG during a response. The NCP states that for a Spill of National Significance in the coastal zone, USCG may name a National Incident Commander who assumes the role of the OSC in communicating with affected parties and coordinating resources at the national level. The NCP further states that coordination will involve the NRT, RRTs, and others as appropriate. However, the NCP does not address how high level officials other than the National Incident Commander can and should participate in such a response."* EPA does have decision-making authority under Subpart J of the NCP. The EPA representative to the RRT must concur on any pre-authorization for the use of chemical agents (such as dispersants, surface washing agents, surface collecting agents, bioremediation agents, and miscellaneous oil spill agents) for any oil spill. The EPA representative to the RRT must also concur on the use of chemical agents for spill situations not addressed by preauthorization plans. Finally, 40CFR300.323(b) addresses the role of EPA senior officials in responding to a Spill of National Significance which provides EPA a concurrence role; 40 CFR 300.323(b) provides that the Administrator may name a senior Agency official to assist in strategic coordination.

10. Page 16. *"It was unclear in our review what responders based the 15,000-gallon limit upon, but the Addendum sought to limit dispersant use and require more documentation because of concerns about ongoing dispersant applications at such large volumes."* The gallon limit was based on a 75% reduction in the total volume of dispersant used.

11. Page 17, *"Rather than EPA's involvement occurring though the RRT and NRT as would happen in a typical response under the NCP, senior EPA officials became involved in daily surface dispersant decisions....Key staff in Region 6, including EPA's representative to the Region 6 RRT and staff involved in the response, said they did not have the authority to approve dispersant applications."* The text should go on to point that out the RRT representative was heavily involved in the decision-making process, and that the decision-making process included the RRT and the NRT members. Senior Agency officials in Area Command, in consultation with EPA's representatives in the Incident Command, gave concurrence to the FOSC.

12. Page 17, *"The concurrence process in place for surface dispersants inherently created delays as EPA elevated decisions to the OSWER Assistant Administrator and, at times, to the Administrator."* We are unclear on the support in the record that delays occurred or were inherent given the frequent and ready communication within the Agency. Timely decisions were made given the magnitude of dispersant use.

> See Appendix D, Note 4, for OIG Response.

13. Page 18, *"OSWER agrees that the NCP needs additional clarity on the roles and responsibilities of various agencies, as well as coordination and communication, for responding to a Spill of National Significance."* The statement needs to be clarified to, "OSWER supports clarification of roles for SONS in NRT guidance. Further evaluation of changes to the NCP is on-going."

14. Page 18, *"EPA increased its involvement in the Deepwater Horizon oil spill over the role envisioned for the Agency in the NCP for deepwater spills."* EPA increased its involvement because the amount of dispersant used and the way in which it was applied (subsea) was unprecedented. EPA does not view this involvement as outside the role envisioned by the NCP for deepwater spills since, as stated above, EPA must concur on the use of dispersants in all spills.

Recommendations

As stated earlier, EPA generally agrees with most of OIG's recommendations. Work is already under way to address most of the recommendations. However, EPA needs to modify recommendation 5 and 7, as noted below, to agree with these recommendations as well.

For recommendation 5, EPA has developed training on roles and responsibilities for large scale events. The NRT is also addressing lessons learned. As such, we propose revising recommendation 5 to state, "*Develop training for a Spill of National Significance event that clarifies roles and responsibilities for high-level agency officials. Review the response and work with federal partners to address lessons learned.*"

For recommendation 7, we want to clarify that the proposed rule may ask for comment on the manufacturer being responsible for tracking production capacities since this would not be an EPA responsibility.

OIG Evaluation of OSWER's Response

General Comments

OSWER generally agreed with our report recommendations. We revised our report text as appropriate based on OSWER's response to our draft report, most notably to note the unprecedented nature of the Deepwater Horizon oil spill and to clarify that we did not intend to imply that EPA's support to the USCG was inadequate or that decisions were inappropriate or inconsistent with the NCP. The following points pertain to those remarks in OSWER's response that required OIG rebuttal based on facts obtained through our review.

Note 1 – Response to Chapter 3 Comment 1

We changed our final report to read, "While we agree that EPA's Administrator retains delegated authority, we found that EPA's involvement of senior Agency officials, in addition to the RRT representative, created confusion on roles and responsibilities. EPA's involvement in dispersant decisions was primarily due to USCG's request given concerns surrounding the use of dispersants and subsea application." We understand that EPA felt it necessary to structure this concurrence process in light of the unprecedented nature of the spill; however, the EPA representative to the RRT stated that they did not have the decision making authority within EPA. Applying lessons learned from this response would help clarify roles and responsibilities of senior Agency officials alongside those of responders identified in the NCP (e.g., RRT representatives).

Note 2 – Response to Chapter 3 Comment 5

We added text to clarify these statements. Our three bulleted examples meant to demonstrate events that should trigger updates to contingency plans, regardless of whether or not dispersants were used. We agree with OSWER that dispersants were not used in the 2002 Gulf of Mexico Spill of National Significance exercise, but the lessons learned document from the exercise considers the use of dispersants a national issue and assigned EPA and the USCG to address the shortfalls of dispersants. Additionally, Hurricanes Katrina and Rita caused a great deal of damage in the Gulf of Mexico to oil facilities, yet deepwater contingency plans were not updated to account for simultaneous events and/or the extensive damage that they caused.

Note 3 – Response to Chapter 3 Comment 6

In addition to spilling 3.3 million barrels of oil and lasting over 10 months, between 1 and 2.5 million gallons of dispersants were applied in response to the Ixtoc I spill. Even though this spill occurred prior to OPA and the Area Contingency Plan, the Ixtoc I spill duration and amount of dispersants was not considered when drafting either of these documents. We understand that the Deepwater Horizon oil spill was unprecedented in many ways, yet the historic Ixtoc I spill could have been taken into consideration when developing planning documents.

Note 4 – Response to Chapter 3 Comment 12

As OSWER noted in its chapter 3 comment 7, pre-approval was developed to assure that the FOSC and/or the responsible party has appropriate tools for immediate response to a spill. We noted that the concurrence process developed during the response—wherein EPA escalated decisions to senior Agency officials instead of the RRT representative—created delays. We observed some examples where it took several hours for some dispersant application decisions and noted that these decisions could have been more immediate had EPA's RRT representative been able to make decisions in real time. We understand that this was an unprecedented spill and are not in a position to say decisions were "untimely" given the magnitude of the response. We recognize the value of senior management's decisionmaking and taking responsibility for those decisions. Nevertheless, escalating decisions up the command chain creates delays over decisions made instantly by the RRT representative.

ORD's Response to Draft Report

June 30, 2011

MEMORANDUM

Subject: OIG's Draft Report: *"Revisions Needed to National Contingency Plan Based on Deepwater Horizon Oil Spill,"* Project No. OA-FY10-0221

From: Paul T. Anastas, PhD
Assistant Administrator for Research and Development

To: Melissa M. Heist
Assistant Inspector General for Audit

We have reviewed the Office of Inspector General (OIG) draft audit report: *"Revisions Needed to National Contingency Plan Based on Deepwater Horizon Oil Spill"* (Project No. OA-FY10-0221), dated May 24, 2011. While we are aware that the Office of Solid Waste and Emergency Response (OSWER) is providing a more in-depth response articulating clarifications and concerns with some of the recommendations and findings, this letter is to state ORD's concurrence with the OIG's recommendation to ORD and have already made significant progress toward that end.

The recommendation to "Develop a research plan to address gaps on long-term and environmental effects of dispersants," is one we have already begun to address. We have developed a longer-term research strategy to address gaps specifically related to the health and environmental effects of dispersants, as well as addressing other oil spill-related research needs. Our strategy has been reviewed by the EPA Science Advisory Board and we anticipate publication in Fall 2011.

Our goal is to support the Agency's mission and decision-making through sound science. We appreciate the review by OIG and the opportunity to comment on this report as it pertains to EPA's research program. Should you have any questions, please contact Cindy Sonich-Mullin, National Homeland Security Research Center, ORD at (513) 569-7923 or Norman Adkins, Office of Resources Management and Administration at (919) 541-0872.

Distribution

Office of the Administrator
Assistant Administrator for Solid Waste and Emergency Response
Assistant Administrator for Research and Development
Regional Administrator, Region 6
Agency Followup Official (the CFO)
Agency Followup Coordinator
General Counsel
Associate Administrator for Congressional and Intergovernmental Relations
Associate Administrator for External Affairs and Environmental Education
Director, Office of Regional Operations
Audit Followup Coordinator, Office of Solid Waste and Emergency Response
Audit Followup Coordinator, Office of Research and Development
Audit Followup Coordinator, Region 6
Director, Office of External Affairs, Region 6

www.ingramcontent.com/pod-product-compliance
Lightning Source LLC
Chambersburg PA
CBHW081802170526
45167CB00008B/3290